I0448922

Lifestyle Choices for a Healthier You

Kris Miller

Copyright © 2010 by Kris Miller.

Library of Congress Control Number:		2010909894
ISBN:	Hardcover	978-1-4535-3280-5
	Softcover	978-1-4535-3279-9
	Ebook	978-1-4535-3281-2

All rights reserved. No part of this book may be reproduced or transmitted in any form or by any means, electronic or mechanical, including photocopying, recording, or by any information storage and retrieval system, without permission in writing from the copyright owner.

This book was printed in the United States of America.

To order additional copies of this book, contact:
Xlibris Corporation
1-888-795-4274
www.Xlibris.com
Orders@Xlibris.com
82727

Table of Contents

We all want to get a little healthier, maybe lose some weight, or start an exercise program, but where do we find the time to research all the information available?

The Lifestyle Choices for a Healthier You Program includes information on valuable websites to help start an exercise program, exercises to do at home, nutrition tips, recipes, making healthy choices when eating out and much more.

Also included are 60-day food and exercise journals and an appointment schedule for exercise. Many people find keeping a journal helps them to stay on track and motivated to reach their goals.

The time is now to start making healthy lifestyle changes. With these tools and my assistance, we will change habits, change attitudes and get you on the road to success!

The information contained in this program is provided for general informational purposes only. It is not intended as and should not be relied upon as medical advice. Check with your doctor before starting any diet or exercise program.

Goal Setting for Nutrition

When setting goals for nutrition it is best to take small steps. Whether you are looking to lower blood pressure or cholesterol, lose weight, feel better, or set a better example for your family your goals should take into account both the kinds and amounts of foods you eat.

Ask Yourself Questions

1. What habits do I want to change?
2. Are my goals realistic?
3. How soon do I want to achieve these goals?
4. Was I successful in accomplishing previous goals?
5. If not, what got in the way? And how can I overcome those obstacles or barriers?
6. If I was successful in accomplishing my goal, how can I build on that success and set a new, slightly higher goal?

Be Specific

Instead of setting a long-term goal that may seem very hard to achieve, focus on a few "mini-goals" keeping you motivated to reach the long-term goal.

Examples:

- Eat breakfast three times per week for one month.
- Eat one fruit and one vegetable four times per week over the next four weeks.
- Increase water intake to eight glasses per day by the end of two months.
- Decrease the amount of soft drinks to one per day.

Write It Down

After you've come up with your goals write them down. Putting them on paper may help keep you more committed.

Post your goals somewhere you will see them often—your refrigerator, desk, or anywhere else to keep you motivated.

Food Journaling

A food journal is a great way to help you become aware of what and how much you eat. A journal is a simple technique to help keep you motivated and on track. It's like your own personal coach. It will also provide you with a permanent record of what you are doing and what is working and what is not.

Benefits of Food Journaling

- When it comes down to it, most of us have only a vague idea of how much we consume and our eating patterns. Writing down food items, portions and emotions may help you develop an awareness of existing problem areas and find what triggers are occurring.
- You can identify problem areas, such as excessive portions, frequent snacking or lack of activity you wish to tackle and provide a permanent record of what you did and can also be used for review.
- Once you identify the triggers—you can take steps to correct or replace certain behaviors before reaching for food.
- Use your journal to keep you motivated, monitor your results, and to program yourself for a lifetime of better health and fitness.
- It is a good idea to record your entries as they occur throughout the day, rather than filling it in each night while trying to remember what you ate during the day.
- Record your success and your failures, so you can look back and see what you've done right and what needs improvement.
- You may discover you may not be eating enough, are eating too much or just eating the wrong things.

- It forces you to become aware of what and how much you eat and allows you to look back and see how you are doing.
- They help to plan meals and keep you motivated.
- Many of us are accustomed to eating unconsciously and munching on whatever comes our way or tempts us at the time.
- You become more disciplined with your lifestyle patterns. You will think twice about overeating, skipping meals or missing your workout.

Alternatives to the Gym

Going to the gym is not a necessity. Basically a pair of athletic shoes and some motivation is all you need to get started on making your lifestyle changes.

1. Check your local library for Exercise DVD'S, videos or books that you can check out, which gives you the opportunity to try them before you purchase them. You could also see if friends or neighbors may have some they want to share.

2. Fitness Magazines or Websites have strength training or cardio workouts you can do at home.

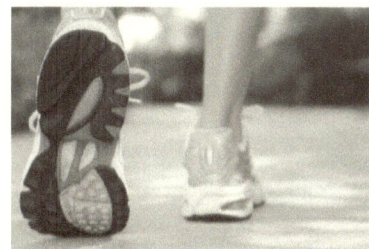

3. Cable stations may offer various types of workouts. With this option you can do them right away or tape them for a later time.

4. Walk around the mall or check with your local high school to see if they offer before or after school walking programs.

5. Pedometers are a great way to track your steps throughout the day. You can start small and set goals to get yourself to where you want to be.

6. If you do not have hand weights available try soup cans or any other type of cans as alternatives.

7. The Wii Fit component of the Wii Video Game System features four main categories to choose from: Strength Training, Aerobics, Yoga and Balance Games. As you spend time exercising, you'll earn Fit Credits that unlock additional exercises and activities within these categories. Wii Fit also tracks the activities you do the most and puts them into the Favorites category.

Goal Setting for Physical Activity

Be sure to set realistic goals when trying to work activity into your daily lifestyle. Activity does not have to take up a lot of time. Many people find they can significantly increase their activity by setting small achievable goals.

Ask Yourself Questions

1. What do I hope to get out of my fitness program?
2. Are my goals realistic?
3. How soon do I want to achieve these goals?
4. Was I successful in accomplishing previous goals?
5. If not, what got in the way? And how can I overcome those obstacles or barriers?
6. If I was successful in accomplishing my goal, how can I further my success and set a new, slightly higher goal?

Be Specific

Instead of setting long-term goals that may seem very hard to achieve, focus on a few "mini-goals" keeping you motivated to reach the long-term goal.

Examples:

- Exercise for at least twenty minutes three times per week.
- Strength train with hand weights two times per week.
- By the end of the week, I will find out about exercise classes offered in my area.

Write It Down

After you've come up with your goals write them down. Putting them on paper will help keep you committed.

Post your goals somewhere you will see them often—your refrigerator, desk or anywhere else that will keep you motivated.

Make a schedule that will be easy for you to follow. Write down the days and times that will work the best for you and by having a routine it may be easier for you to follow and stick with an exercise program.

Make an appointment to exercise and stick to it. We are not likely to cancel appointments such as the doctor or dentist, so why not make the time to exercise and consider it an important appointment too.

Healthy Lifestyle Tips

1. Pre-plan meals and snacks. Taking an hour or so each week to plan meals or cut up fruits and vegetables for snacks may help you stick with healthy eating. When food is available to grab on the go or heat up in a few minutes, it may be easier to stay focused and motivated to make healthy choices.

2. Don't skip meals or snacks as you will be less likely to experience cravings. Most important don't skip breakfast. You haven't eaten since dinner the night before and breakfast helps to jump-start your metabolism for the day, and help with your performance.

3. Eat what you like, otherwise you're going to feel deprived or you may find yourself binging on high-calorie foods and feel bad for straying from the plan. All foods can fit into a well-balanced diet.

4. Pay attention to portions. Serve meals that are already plated and do not put serving bowls on tables. If you have to get up from the table to get seconds you may not want them as much.

5. Don't keep comfort foods in the house. If you eat high-fat or high-calorie foods when bored or stressed, don't keep those items in the house.

6. De-stress your day. Sometimes stress can cause you to eat more. Find activities helping you to relax such as deep breathing exercises, reading, taking a bath, calling a friend or exercising.

7. Vary your exercise activities. Changing up your activities will help avoid exercise burnout. Checking out classes at your local community center or renting an exercise video may add to a walking routine.

8. Plate size. Serve your meals on a small salad plate instead of a dinner plate.

9. Don't eat on the run. Sit-down and take note of what you are eating. It is a good time to focus on what you are eating and how you are feeling and record it in your journal.

10. Don't beat yourself up if you had a bad day in regards to exercise and nutrition. We all slip up at times, but it is important to get right back on track. If you tell yourself your going to get started again next week, it might be hard to get back into your routine.

11. Sometimes starting an exercise program is the hardest part. Start slowly and work yourself up to your goals. You may only be able to work out for five minutes a couple times per week, but it's a start. It may get frustrating at times, but you might also find you really enjoy exercise!

12. You can make exercise enjoyable by listening to a book on tape, or if you have home equipment set it up in an area where you can watch television. Check with a friend or neighbor to see if they would like to join you for walks in the morning or after dinner. Make it fun and enjoy all the benefits you will receive.

13. Don't expect to see results immediately. It will take sometime to adjust to your workouts and to start building muscle. Remember muscle weighs more than fat, so if you are not seeing the numbers drop on the scale as fast as you would expect, it may be because you are gaining muscle.

14. Think about the foods you should be eating, not the ones you feel you should be avoiding.

15. Water is as important as the food you eat. Try to drink at least six to eight glasses per day or 48-64 ounces. If you are currently drinking little or no water, it may be a challenge to get in eight glasses per day. One way to approach this is to fill a half-gallon container with water and put it in the refrigerator. See how much water you can drink throughout the day. Each day start again and

try to drink more than the day before. In no time, you will be drinking eight glasses daily.

16. Learn how to manage your time according to your priorities.

17. Try not to sample food when you're cooking.

18. Eat because you are hungry, not because you're thirsty. A glass of water or juice may be all you need to stop a craving.

19. When you lose weight at a slower pace, you are more likely to keep it off.

20. No matter what eating plan you follow, losing weight boils down to burning more calories than you consume.

21. Drink enough water and cut back on sugary snacks.

22. Eat three small meals and one to two snacks daily.

23. Make one day/evening "cooking" day. Make a casserole or something and freeze individual portions for quick lunches.

24. Look for a distraction when you're fighting a craving. Call a friend, clean the house, put on music and dance, exercise or run an errand. When your mind is occupied with something else, the cravings quickly go away.

25. Stock your pantry with healthy foods.

26. Many people may think of snacking as bad for you, but it doesn't have to be that way. Snacking can be very beneficial to a balanced diet. Healthy snacking may help to improve overall health, curb cravings, fight weight gain, regulate mood, keep your mind alert and give you the energy you need to keep going all day.

27. Strength training exercises, when done properly and through full range of motion, can help to increase a person's flexibility and balance, which may decrease the odds and severity of falls.

These exercises can also be effective in reducing the signs and symptoms of many diseases and chronic conditions. Some examples are: arthritis, obesity, osteoporosis, diabetes and back pain.

28. In a restaurant, start your meal with a salad packed with vegetables to help control hunger and feel satisfied sooner. Order salad dressings on the side, so you are in control of adding as much or little as you want.

29. Use your food budget wisely. For the price of a large bag of chips and a box of cookies, you can buy lots of fruits, vegetables and healthier foods.

30. If you do not enjoy drinking water by itself, add a little fruit or fruit juice to add a little extra flavor. Powder packets such as Propel are also a good choice.

31. Moderation is the key: eat a variety of foods you enjoy, but watch serving sizes.

32. Eat slowly and chew your food well. This allows you to realize you are full before you overeat.

33. Choose foods labeled sodium free, low sodium or reduced sodium.

34. Taste foods before you add salt. Use salt-free seasonings, spices and herbs when cooking and at the table.

35. Decrease your fat and sugar intake and your caloric intake will likely decrease.

36. It is better to have a little something in the morning than skipping breakfast altogether. Start small. If you are not use to eating breakfast begin with yogurt, fruit, or a piece of whole-wheat toast. In a few days try to add more foods. If that does not work, just stick with what you are doing.

37. Eating fiber is one of the easiest and best things you can do for your health.

38. One of the benefits of fiber is it helps you to maintain a healthy weight. High-fiber foods tend to be lower in fat, and they also fill you up more.

39. Some factors to consider when getting started and keeping at an exercise program are: "What do I like to do?", "Do I want to exercise alone or with others?" and "What are my exercise goals and how do I plan to reach them?"

40. Healthier fast food choices might include: regular single patty hamburger without the mayo or cheese, grilled chicken sandwich, garden salad with grilled chicken and low-fat dressing, baked potato or a side salad.

Appendix

Summaries of Websites

Listed below are a few of the websites I have used to find information in regards to health, nutrition, fitness and weight loss.

I.   My Pyramid: www.mypyramid.gov

Topics Covered:

My Pyramid Basics
-   Inside the Pyramid
-   Tips and Resources
-   Print Materials
-   Answers to Questions

Interactive Tools
-   My Pyramid Plan
-   Menu Planner
-   My Pyramid Tracker—Assess your food intake and physical activity

Steps to a Healthier Weight
-   Dietary Guidelines

Inside the Pyramid
-   Gives information regarding grains, vegetables, fruits, milk, meat and beans, oil, and discretionary calories.
-   What is included in each group?
-   How much is needed?
-   Health benefits and nutrients.
-   Tips to help you eat foods in these groups.

Physical Activity
-   What is physical activity?
-   Why is it important?
-   How much is needed?
-   Tips for increasing physical activity.

II. ACE Fitness: www.acefitness.org

This website contains an exercise library that gives step by step instructions on exercises for the abs, butt and hips, legs, shoulders, back, chest, arms and also full-body workouts.

Healthy recipes for appetizers, salads, main dishes, desserts and baked goods, beverages, soups and stews, side dishes, sauces and dressings.

Also included are health and fitness tips.

III. American Dietetic Association: www.eatright.org

This website has a section entitled For the Public. Some of the topics covered are as follows:

Nutrition for Life
Healthy Weight
Food & Nutrition
Disease Management and Prevention

IV. Healthy Dining Finder: www.healthydiningfinder.com

Restaurants featured on this site have joined the Healthy Dining Program because they have a sincere interest in offering their customers healthier choices.

Sections covered:
About the restaurants
Nutrition Criteria
Nutrition 101: Topics covered: Fruits and veggies, whole grains, calories, fat, cholesterol, sodium, carbohydrates and proteins.

VI. Additional Resources:

American Heart Association
    www.americanheart.org

Fruits and Veggies More Matters
    www.fruitsandveggiesmorematters.org

Prevention Magazine
    www.prevention.com

Others:
    www.foodfit.com
    www.nutrition.gov
    www.cookinglight.com

Weekly Wrap-Up

> What were some positives of your week?

> Did you exercise three times this week? Did you say 'no' to dessert at a restaurant or party? Did you drink at least six to eight glasses of water per day?

> Writing down your positive actions will help you to continue them in the future.

> What were some challenges?

> Did you eat too many chips or cookies after a bad day at work? Did you miss a couple of days of exercise at the beginning of the week and therefore decided not to do any?

> Challenges will occur, so this will be a good time to come up with ways to handle things differently if these situations should happen again.

> Is there anything you would like to do differently next week? Add more exercise, try a new recipe, or increase your servings of fruits and vegetables?

Short Term Goals

Nutrition

Week 1
Eat breakfast at least
3 days per week

Week 2
Increase water intake to
at least 6 glasses/day

Weeks 3
Have a salad or vegetable
with dinner

Week 4
Cut back to eating fast food
to only one time/week

Physical Activity

Week 1
I will walk 15 minutes
3 days per week

Week 2
By the end of the week I will talk to
my friend about exercising with me
a couple of times/week

Week 3
I will check out an exercise
video from the library
to add variety to my exercise

Week 4
Add strength training with hand
weights at least once/week

Long Term Goals

Nutrition

6 Month

Eat at least 2 fruits and 2 vegetables per day

12 Months

Bring cholesterol down before next doctor's visit by changing
my eating habits

Physical Activity

6 Months

I will walk at least 5 days per week for 30 minutes

12 Month

I will enter a 5K walk/run

Exercise Appointment Calendar

Sun	Mon	Tues	Wed	Th	Fri	Sat
	1	2	3	4	5	6
	Walk 15 minutes at lunch	20 minute strength training video at home	Walk 15 minutes at lunch	20 minute strength training video at home	Walk 15 minute at lunch	Bike ride with family
7	8	9	10	11	12	13
	Walk 20 minutes before work	20 minute pilate video	Walk 20 minutes after work	20 minute pilate video	Walk 20 minutes before work	Nature walk with family
14	15	16				

SAMPLE

Food Journal

Day 1

	Breakfast	Snack	Lunch	Snack	Dinner	Snack
Food Items	Milk Oatmeal Blueberries	1 Yogurt	Salad w/Chicken Lite Dressing 2 Rye Crisps	12 Almonds Apple	Fish Brown Rice Steamed Vegetables Milk	5 Whole Wheat Crackers
Time	7:00 AM	10:00 AM	12:30 PM	3:30 PM	6:00 PM	8:00 PM
Feeling	Hungry	Bored	Hungry	Tired	Hungry & Family Time	Something to do

Water ☑ ☑ ☑ ☑ ☑ ☑ ☑ ☑

Activity	Time
Walked steps to doctors Appointment	9:30 AM
15 Minute walk at lunch	1:00 PM
Played ball with kids	2:00 PM
Family walk after dinner	6:30 PM

Notes Found a new recipe to try for dinner tomorrow night

_____

_____

Health Tip
When developing an exercise plan make sure to have a clear vision of what you want from exercise, develop a plan of action, and identify tools and support systems to put your plan into action.

Notes:

* Looked at Fitness Magazine in doctor's office and saw a video called Pilates for Beginners. Will check to see if they have it at the library or on Amazon.com

* While visiting a friend we enjoyed smoothies. I asked her for the recipe:

Bright Eyed Strawberry Banana Boost
1 cup low fat strawberry yogurt
1 cup frozen strawberries
1 1/2 bananas
3/4 milk

* Looking for information on calorie counting. A co-worker suggested looking on Amazon.com for some different options.

* Reminder: Check email to see if coupons came from Healthy Dining Finder

Short Term Goals

Nutrition

Week 1

_____

_____

_____

Week 2

_____

_____

_____

Week 3

_____

_____

_____

Week 4

_____

_____

_____

Physical Activity

Week 1

_____

_____

_____

Week 2

_____

_____

_____

Week 3

_____

_____

_____

Week 4

_____

_____

_____

Long Term Goals

Nutrition

6 Month

_____

_____

_____

12 Month

_____

_____

_____

Physical Activity

6 Month

_____

_____

_____

12 Month

_____

_____

_____

Exercise Appointment Calendar

Sun	Mon	Tues	Wed	Th	Fri	Sat

Notes:

Day 1   Food Journal

	Breakfast	Snack	Lunch	Snack	Dinner	Snack
Food Items						
Time						
Feeling						

Water ☐ ☐ ☐ ☐ ☐ ☐ ☐ ☐

Activity	Time

Notes _____

_____

Health Tip
The key to attaining better health is to develop a strategy to incorporate healthy decisions into daily life.

Day 2 Food Journal

	Breakfast	Snack	Lunch	Snack	Dinner	Snack
Food Items						
Time						
Feeling						

Water ☐ ☐ ☐ ☐ ☐ ☐ ☐ ☐

Activity	Time

Notes _____

_____

Health Tip
When developing an exercise plan make sure to have a clear vision of what you want from exercise, develop a plan of action, and identify tools and support systems to put your plan into action.

Day 3   Food Journal

	Breakfast	Snack	Lunch	Snack	Dinner	Snack
Food Items						
Time						
Feeling						

Water ☐ ☐ ☐ ☐ ☐ ☐ ☐ ☐

Activity	Time

Notes _____

_____

Health Tip

Starting the day with breakfast, especially a breakfast high in fiber, may help control calorie intake the rest of the day.

Day 4   **Food Journal**

	Breakfast	Snack	Lunch	Snack	Dinner	Snack
Food Items						
Time						
Feeling						

Water ☐ ☐ ☐ ☐ ☐ ☐ ☐ ☐

Activity	Time

Notes _____

_____

Health Tip
You can always find an excuse for not eating right or exercising - use excuses and you will never achieve the kind of health and fitness you are looking to attain.

Day 5   Food Journal

	Breakfast	Snack	Lunch	Snack	Dinner	Snack
Food Items						
Time						
Feeling						

Water ☐ ☐ ☐ ☐ ☐ ☐ ☐ ☐

Activity	Time

Notes _____

_____

Health Tip
Bring a bottle of water with you always and keep drinking throughout the day.

Day 6 — Food Journal

	Breakfast	Snack	Lunch	Snack	Dinner	Snack
Food Items						
Time						
Feeling						

Water ☐ ☐ ☐ ☐ ☐ ☐ ☐ ☐

Activity	Time

Notes _____

_____

Health Tip

Set lifestyle goals - not weight loss goals. Commitment to eating healthy foods does lead to healthy weight loss - gradually.

Day 7 Food Journal

	Breakfast	Snack	Lunch	Snack	Dinner	Snack
Food Items						
Time						
Feeling						

Water ☐ ☐ ☐ ☐ ☐ ☐ ☐ ☐

Activity	Time

Notes _____

_____

Health Tip
Don't fall into bad habits on weekends. Many people will follow a strict diet on weekdays only to fall back into eating more (unhealthy) on the weekends as reward for being good all week.

Day 8   **Food Journal**

	Breakfast	Snack	Lunch	Snack	Dinner	Snack
Food Items						
Time						
Feeling						

Water ☐ ☐ ☐ ☐ ☐ ☐ ☐ ☐

Activity	Time

Notes _____

_____

Health Tip
If you feel your energy dropping in the middle of the day, get up and go for a short walk or do some other physical activity. This will re-energize you instead of reaching for caffeine or sugary snacks.

Day 9   Food Journal

	Breakfast	Snack	Lunch	Snack	Dinner	Snack
Food Items						
Time						
Feeling						

Water ☐ ☐ ☐ ☐ ☐ ☐ ☐ ☐

Activity	Time

Notes _____

_____

Health Tip
Learn to laugh. Laughter is a powerful medicine that helps us develop better perspectives during stressful situations.

Day 10   Food Journal

	Breakfast	Snack	Lunch	Snack	Dinner	Snack
Food Items						
Time						
Feeling						

Water ☐ ☐ ☐ ☐ ☐ ☐ ☐ ☐

Activity	Time

Notes _____

_____

Health Tip

A good way to enjoy the food you eat and to avoid overeating is to pay attention to the present moment. Be conscious of what you are eating and how you are feeling as you are doing it. Choose to eat foods that you enjoy and will provide nourishment for your body.

Day 11   Food Journal

	Breakfast	Snack	Lunch	Snack	Dinner	Snack
Food Items						
Time						
Feeling						

Water ☐ ☐ ☐ ☐ ☐ ☐ ☐ ☐

Activity	Time

Notes _____

_____

Health Tip
A healthy diet is like jogging. Practice a few times and it will come naturally.

Day 12 Food Journal

	Breakfast	Snack	Lunch	Snack	Dinner	Snack
Food Items						
Time						
Feeling						

Water ☐ ☐ ☐ ☐ ☐ ☐ ☐ ☐

Activity	Time

Notes _____

_____

Health Tip
Research shows that eating a wide variety of fruits and vegetables protects you against cancer, heart disease and the effects of aging. Experiment with a variety of brightly colored fruits and vegetables and think of the rainbow when putting together a salad or vegetable tray.

Day 13   Food Journal

	Breakfast	Snack	Lunch	Snack	Dinner	Snack
Food Items						
Time						
Feeling						

Water ☐ ☐ ☐ ☐ ☐ ☐ ☐ ☐

Activity	Time

Notes _____

_____

Health Tip
Focus on what you want in life. If you have trouble discovering what you want, just evaluate what you do not want and change it to what you want. For example, if you do not want to be overweight, change it to I want to be fit, healthy and at my ideal weight.

Day 14   **Food Journal**

	Breakfast	Snack	Lunch	Snack	Dinner	Snack
Food Items						
Time						
Feeling						

Water ☐ ☐ ☐ ☐ ☐ ☐ ☐ ☐

Activity	Time

Notes _____

_____

Health Tip

A key to getting in shape is determination and consistency. Notice how your body responds to exercise and truly enjoy the benefits of exercise. The more you focus on the benefits the easier it will be to motivate yourself to stick with your fitness plan.

Day 15   Food Journal

	Breakfast	Snack	Lunch	Snack	Dinner	Snack
Food Items						
Time						
Feeling						

Water ☐ ☐ ☐ ☐ ☐ ☐ ☐ ☐

Activity	Time

Notes _____

_____

Health Tip
To truly achieve vibrant health, you must know why you want it. Take time today to write down at least twenty reasons why vibrant health is important to you and review your list everyday.

Day 16   Food Journal

	Breakfast	Snack	Lunch	Snack	Dinner	Snack
Food Items						
Time						
Feeling						

Water ☐ ☐ ☐ ☐ ☐ ☐ ☐ ☐

Activity	Time

Notes _____

_____

Health Tip
Deep breathing is a great way to calm yourself and energize your body. A good deep breathing technique is to sit comfortably, breathe in for five counts, hold your breath for five counts, and breathe out for five counts. Do this 1-2 minutes.

Day 17   **Food Journal**

	Breakfast	Snack	Lunch	Snack	Dinner	Snack
Food Items						
Time						
Feeling						

Water ☐ ☐ ☐ ☐ ☐ ☐ ☐ ☐

Activity	Time

Notes _____

_____

Health Tip
DO NOT use the fact that you are not 100% physically fit as an excuse not to exercise. In fact, in most cases, the only way to get closer to that 100% is to follow a consistent fitness program.

Day 18   Food Journal

	Breakfast	Snack	Lunch	Snack	Dinner	Snack
Food Items						
Time						
Feeling						

Water ☐ ☐ ☐ ☐ ☐ ☐ ☐ ☐

Activity	Time

Notes _____

_____

Health Tip
Persistence makes up for lack of skill in anything you choose to master, especially when you are working towards your fitness goals.

Day 19

Food Journal

	Breakfast	Snack	Lunch	Snack	Dinner	Snack
Food Items						
Time						
Feeling						

Water ☐ ☐ ☐ ☐ ☐ ☐ ☐ ☐

Activity	Time

Notes _____

_____

Health Tip

Research shows that making small changes can add up to a big difference in your health over time. By doing a little every week to improve your health, you will notice a big improvement in your overall sense of well-being.

Day 20

Food Journal

	Breakfast	Snack	Lunch	Snack	Dinner	Snack
Food Items						
Time						
Feeling						

Water ☐ ☐ ☐ ☐ ☐ ☐ ☐ ☐

Activity	Time

Notes _____

Health Tip

The College of Alumni Health study has shown that if you become and remain active you will live longer, look better, have more vitality, think more clearly and sleep better.

Day 21　　　　　　　　　　　　Food Journal

	Breakfast	Snack	Lunch	Snack	Dinner	Snack
Food Items						
Time						
Feeling						

Water ☐ ☐ ☐ ☐ ☐ ☐ ☐ ☐

Activity	Time

Notes _____

_____

Health Tip
As you set health and wellness goals, write down specifically what you want to achieve and when you want to achieve these goals. Read your goals daily so they become part of you.

Day 22   Food Journal

	Breakfast	Snack	Lunch	Snack	Dinner	Snack
Food Items						
Time						
Feeling						

Water ☐ ☐ ☐ ☐ ☐ ☐ ☐ ☐

Activity	Time

Notes _____

_____

Health Tip
To be truly healthy it is important to be good to yourself. Treat yourself with love and respect.

Day 23 Food Journal

	Breakfast	Snack	Lunch	Snack	Dinner	Snack
Food Items						
Time						
Feeling						

Water ☐ ☐ ☐ ☐ ☐ ☐ ☐ ☐

Activity	Time

Notes _____

_____

Health Tip
If you are having trouble motivating yourself to exercise, enlist the help of a friend. When you are accountable to someone else, you are more likely to follow through with your exercise plan.

Day 24   **Food Journal**

	Breakfast	Snack	Lunch	Snack	Dinner	Snack
Food Items						
Time						
Feeling						

Water ☐ ☐ ☐ ☐ ☐ ☐ ☐ ☐

Activity	Time

Notes _____

_____

Health Tip
Children learn best by example instead of lecturing them about healthy eating. As parents improve their diet and focus on physical activity, it will be easier to influence their children to live a healthier lifestyle.

Day 25   Food Journal

	Breakfast	Snack	Lunch	Snack	Dinner	Snack
Food Items						
Time						
Feeling						

Water ☐ ☐ ☐ ☐ ☐ ☐ ☐ ☐

Activity	Time

Notes _____

_____

Health Tip
A great way to motivate yourself to exercise first thing in the morning is to lay out your exercise clothes and prepare a water bottle the night before. When you wake up in the morning you will see the exercise clothes and be inspired to get moving.

Day 26 Food Journal

	Breakfast	Snack	Lunch	Snack	Dinner	Snack
Food Items						
Time						
Feeling						

Water ☐ ☐ ☐ ☐ ☐ ☐ ☐ ☐

Activity	Time

Notes _____

_____

Health Tip
Be realistic with your goals. If they are too hard to accomplish, you may get frustrated and never meet them.

Day 27   Food Journal

	Breakfast	Snack	Lunch	Snack	Dinner	Snack
Food Items						
Time						
Feeling						

Water ☐ ☐ ☐ ☐ ☐ ☐ ☐ ☐

Activity	Time

Notes _____

_____

Health Tip
People who skip meals generally have a slower metabolism than those who do not because depriving the body of food causes its metabolism to slow down.

Day28   Food Journal

	Breakfast	Snack	Lunch	Snack	Dinner	Snack
Food Items						
Time						
Feeling						

Water ☐ ☐ ☐ ☐ ☐ ☐ ☐ ☐

Activity	Time

Notes _____

_____

Health Tip
Soft drinks are the number one contributor of sugar in the American diet. A twelve ounce can of regular soda contributes ten teaspoons of sugar alone.

Day 29　　　　　　　　　　　**Food Journal**

	Breakfast	Snack	Lunch	Snack	Dinner	Snack
Food Items						
Time						
Feeling						

Water ☐ ☐ ☐ ☐ ☐ ☐ ☐ ☐

Activity	Time

Notes _____

_____

Health Tip
Regular exercise is also effective in preventing bone loss that can contribute to osteoporosis later in life.

Day 30   Food Journal

	Breakfast	Snack	Lunch	Snack	Dinner	Snack
Food Items						
Time						
Feeling						

Water ☐ ☐ ☐ ☐ ☐ ☐ ☐ ☐

Activity	Time

Notes _____

_____

Health Tip
Shop the outer perimeter of your store for the freshest and most nutritious food choices.

Day 31   Food Journal

	Breakfast	Snack	Lunch	Snack	Dinner	Snack
Food Items						
Time						
Feeling						

Water ☐ ☐ ☐ ☐ ☐ ☐ ☐ ☐

Activity	Time

Notes _____

_____

Health Tip
Muscle weighs more than fat, so building up muscle can initially add several pounds rather than taking them off, but in time this will reverse.

Day 32 Food Journal

	Breakfast	Snack	Lunch	Snack	Dinner	Snack
Food Items						
Time						
Feeling						

Water ☐ ☐ ☐ ☐ ☐ ☐ ☐ ☐

Activity	Time

Notes _____

_____

Health Tip
Sit down whenever you eat, whether it is a snack or meal. Sit down and take note of what you are eating. In other words, no eating on the run or standing in front of the refrigerator.

Day 33   Food Journal

	Breakfast	Snack	Lunch	Snack	Dinner	Snack
Food Items						
Time						
Feeling						

Water ☐ ☐ ☐ ☐ ☐ ☐ ☐ ☐

Activity	Time

Notes _____

_____

Health Tip
Focus on your successes. Concentrate on your accomplishments rather than on your failures. When you put too much attention on where you have failed, you lose track of where you are going.

Day 34 Food Journal

	Breakfast	Snack	Lunch	Snack	Dinner	Snack
Food Items						
Time						
Feeling						

Water ☐ ☐ ☐ ☐ ☐ ☐ ☐ ☐

Activity	Time

Notes _____

_____

Health Tip
There is something to be gained from every challenge you face.

Day 35   Food Journal

	Breakfast	Snack	Lunch	Snack	Dinner	Snack
Food Items						
Time						
Feeling						

Water ☐ ☐ ☐ ☐ ☐ ☐ ☐ ☐

Activity	Time

Notes _____

_____

Health Tip

Exercise is essential to becoming healthy. If you have not exercised regularly, build your activity level slow and steady until it becomes a habit.

Day 36 Food Journal

	Breakfast	Snack	Lunch	Snack	Dinner	Snack
Food Items						
Time						
Feeling						

Water ☐ ☐ ☐ ☐ ☐ ☐ ☐ ☐

Activity	Time

Notes _____

_____

Health Tip
Being aware of how you want to feel in any activity makes it more likely that you will perform well and enjoy the activity, which makes it a positive experience.

Day 37   Food Journal

	Breakfast	Snack	Lunch	Snack	Dinner	Snack
Food Items						
Time						
Feeling						

Water ☐ ☐ ☐ ☐ ☐ ☐ ☐ ☐

Activity	Time

Notes _____

_____

Health Tip
Fun, joy and laughter create health. If what you are doing is not bringing you joy, find something else that will.

Day 38   **Food Journal**

	Breakfast	Snack	Lunch	Snack	Dinner	Snack
Food Items						
Time						
Feeling						

Water ☐ ☐ ☐ ☐ ☐ ☐ ☐ ☐

Activity	Time

Notes _____

_____

Health Tip
Experiment with new foods and physical activity to keep things interesting.

Day 39   Food Journal

	Breakfast	Snack	Lunch	Snack	Dinner	Snack
Food Items						
Time						
Feeling						

Water ☐ ☐ ☐ ☐ ☐ ☐ ☐ ☐

Activity	Time

Notes _____

_____

Health Tip
If you come home from work feeling tired, instead of grabbing a snack or watching TV, break a sweat. A few minutes of vigorous exercise will make you feel better and more energetic.

Day 40　　　　　　　　　　　**Food Journal**

	Breakfast	Snack	Lunch	Snack	Dinner	Snack
Food Items						
Time						
Feeling						

Water ☐ ☐ ☐ ☐ ☐ ☐ ☐ ☐

Activity	Time

Notes _____

_____

Health Tip
If you are interested in lifelong weight management and eating a healthy diet, eat consciously and purposely.

Day 41   Food Journal

	Breakfast	Snack	Lunch	Snack	Dinner	Snack
Food Items						
Time						
Feeling						

Water ☐ ☐ ☐ ☐ ☐ ☐ ☐ ☐

Activity	Time

Notes _____

_____

Health Tip
As you accomplish your health goals, continue setting new goals to motivate you towards optimal fitness and well-being.

Day 42 **Food Journal**

	Breakfast	Snack	Lunch	Snack	Dinner	Snack
Food Items						
Time						
Feeling						

Water ☐ ☐ ☐ ☐ ☐ ☐ ☐ ☐

Activity	Time

Notes _____

_____

Health Tip
Practice leaving just one thing on your plate if you are interested in losing weight.

Day 43   Food Journal

	Breakfast	Snack	Lunch	Snack	Dinner	Snack
Food Items						
Time						
Feeling						

Water ☐ ☐ ☐ ☐ ☐ ☐ ☐ ☐

Activity	Time

Notes _____

_____

Health Tip
An excellent way to motivate yourself to achieve your goals is to write them down.
Post your goals where you will see them often.

Day 44   Food Journal

	Breakfast	Snack	Lunch	Snack	Dinner	Snack
Food Items						
Time						
Feeling						

Water ☐ ☐ ☐ ☐ ☐ ☐ ☐ ☐

Activity	Time

Notes _____

_____

Health Tip
Strength training at least twice weekly will increase your metabolism and increase your potential to burn fat and build muscle mass.

Day 45   Food Journal

	Breakfast	Snack	Lunch	Snack	Dinner	Snack
Food Items						
Time						
Feeling						

Water ☐ ☐ ☐ ☐ ☐ ☐ ☐ ☐

Activity	Time

Notes _____

_____

Health Tip
If you experience a craving for unhealthy food, distract yourself for ten minutes. Often you will find once you get busy doing another activity, the craving will pass.

Day 46　　　　　　　　　　　　Food Journal

	Breakfast	Snack	Lunch	Snack	Dinner	Snack
Food Items						
Time						
Feeling						

Water ☐ ☐ ☐ ☐ ☐ ☐ ☐ ☐

Activity	Time

Notes _____

_____

Health Tip
A study published in the American Journal of Preventative Medicine found that people who kept food diaries lost twice as much weight as those who did not.

Day 47   **Food Journal**

	Breakfast	Snack	Lunch	Snack	Dinner	Snack
Food Items						
Time						
Feeling						

Water ☐ ☐ ☐ ☐ ☐ ☐ ☐ ☐

Activity	Time

Notes _____

_____

Health Tip
A sound nutrition and exercise plan is among the most important factors in reducing stress.

Day 48 Food Journal

	Breakfast	Snack	Lunch	Snack	Dinner	Snack
Food Items						
Time						
Feeling						

Water ☐ ☐ ☐ ☐ ☐ ☐ ☐ ☐

Activity	Time

Notes _____

_____

Health Tip
Plan your diet on a weekly basis, laying out a general well-balanced menu. Planning will help you around the trap of impulsive food buying.

Day 49   Food Journal

	Breakfast	Snack	Lunch	Snack	Dinner	Snack
Food Items						
Time						
Feeling						

Water ☐ ☐ ☐ ☐ ☐ ☐ ☐ ☐

Activity	Time

Notes _____

_____

Health Tip
If you find it difficult to exercise for thirty minutes or more each day, just do five or ten minute intervals. Often you will find it difficult to quit once you get started.

Day 50 Food Journal

	Breakfast	Snack	Lunch	Snack	Dinner	Snack
Food Items						
Time						
Feeling						

Water ☐ ☐ ☐ ☐ ☐ ☐ ☐ ☐

Activity	Time

Notes _____

_____

Health Tip

It is natural to be healthy. Our body does whatever it can to be in a state of health. If you support your body with health promoting choices, your body will respond.

Day 51   Food Journal

	Breakfast	Snack	Lunch	Snack	Dinner	Snack
Food Items						
Time						
Feeling						

Water ☐ ☐ ☐ ☐ ☐ ☐ ☐ ☐

Activity	Time

Notes _____

_____

Health Tip
Grilling is an excellent way to prepare almost any meat or vegetable. It is a fast, easy and tasty way to create a lowfat meal.

Day 52　　　　　　　　　　　　Food Journal

	Breakfast	Snack	Lunch	Snack	Dinner	Snack
Food Items						
Time						
Feeling						

Water ☐ ☐ ☐ ☐ ☐ ☐ ☐ ☐

Activity	Time

Notes _____

_____

Health Tip
To make exercise more enjoyable, focus on all the benefits such as increased energy, weight loss, stress reduction and increased metabolism.

Day 53

Food Journal

	Breakfast	Snack	Lunch	Snack	Dinner	Snack
Food Items						
Time						
Feeling						

Water ☐ ☐ ☐ ☐ ☐ ☐ ☐ ☐

Activity	Time

Notes _____

_____

Health Tip
To curb your hunger before and between meals, snack on low calorie, high water content vegetables such as greens, carrots, tomatoes and cucumbers.

Day 54 Food Journal

	Breakfast	Snack	Lunch	Snack	Dinner	Snack
Food Items						
Time						
Feeling						

Water ☐ ☐ ☐ ☐ ☐ ☐ ☐ ☐

Activity	Time

Notes _____

Health Tip
A recent study found that strength training boosts your metabolism and fat burning capabilities for up to two days after a workout.

Day 55 Food Journal

	Breakfast	Snack	Lunch	Snack	Dinner	Snack
Food Items						
Time						
Feeling						

Water ☐ ☐ ☐ ☐ ☐ ☐ ☐ ☐

Activity	Time

Notes _____

_____

Health Tip
Research has found that combining a healthful diet with aerobic exercise can lower LDL cholesterol by up to twenty points.

Day 56　　　　　　　　　　**Food Journal**

	Breakfast	Snack	Lunch	Snack	Dinner	Snack
Food Items						
Time						
Feeling						

Water ☐ ☐ ☐ ☐ ☐ ☐ ☐ ☐

Activity	Time

Notes _____

_____

Health Tip
Recognize any small improvements in your health and wellness. Celebrate any progress you achieve to motivate yourself for further success.

Day 57   Food Journal

	Breakfast	Snack	Lunch	Snack	Dinner	Snack
Food Items						
Time						
Feeling						

Water ☐ ☐ ☐ ☐ ☐ ☐ ☐ ☐

Activity	Time

Notes _____

_____

Health Tip
Motivation is what gets you started and habit is what keeps you going.

Day 58   Food Journal

	Breakfast	Snack	Lunch	Snack	Dinner	Snack
Food Items						
Time						
Feeling						

Water ☐ ☐ ☐ ☐ ☐ ☐ ☐ ☐

Activity	Time

Notes _____

_____

Health Tip
Think about what to eat rather than what not to eat.

Day 59 Food Journal

	Breakfast	Snack	Lunch	Snack	Dinner	Snack
Food Items						
Time						
Feeling						

Water ☐ ☐ ☐ ☐ ☐ ☐ ☐ ☐

Activity	Time

Notes _____

_____

Health Tip
Whatever type of exercise you decide on the two important factors are that you enjoy the exercise and that you do it regularly.

Day 60   Food Journal

	Breakfast	Snack	Lunch	Snack	Dinner	Snack
Food Items						
Time						
Feeling						

Water ☐ ☐ ☐ ☐ ☐ ☐ ☐ ☐

Activity	Time

Notes _____

_____

Health Tip
Every new day brings with it new possibilities.

www.ingramcontent.com/pod-product-compliance
Lightning Source LLC
Chambersburg PA
CBHW030412290526
45785CB00004B/1980